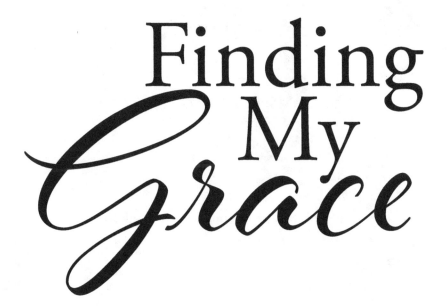

Finding My Grace

KATE CERNY

NEWMAN SPRINGS PUBLISHING
320 Broad Street
Red Bank, NJ 07701

First originally published by Newman Springs Publishing 2021

Cover Photo Credit
Danielle Finder
daniellefinderphoto.pixieset.com

ISBN 978-1-63692-480-9 (Paperback)
ISBN 978-1-63692-481-6 (Digital)

Printed in the United States of America

To Mama and Dad, "thank you" just does not seem like enough.

We all have a voice inside our heads that critiques our actions and words. I refer to this as the "inner Bully." Learning to silence or change the character of that voice is difficult work. I have embarked on a journey to do just that, not just for myself but for others. It is not that I am somehow gifted or enlightened, but through my life's experiences, I have been forced to make radical changes; and controlling my Bully has been the biggest.

FOREWORD

I'm so honored to write this foreword: Kate stole my heart with her zest for life.

We met on the island of Oahu, HI. Our first meeting was a beach walk on the North Shore where I met the dogs, Moe and Albert. As the walk and conversation continued, I knew the three of them were put in my life for a reason. The picturesque scenery and the brilliantly colored sunsets complemented many of our Beach House dinner dates. Looking back at our courtship, it was perfect.

We enjoyed our time on the island while Kate was waiting for her ranch to sell and I was finishing up my Air Force career. In our off-time, we spent combing the beach for colored sea glass for our collection jar and figuring out our life. It was a gift to finally know the inner workings of a survivor and hear my beautiful future wife's story. We clicked and lived each day to the fullest.

As It turned out, we had both overcame a life threatening disease. I've come to find that when a person is faced with their demise, it WILL change an outlook on life. We both totally connected because of our outlook; tomorrow IS NOT guaranteed for anyone. Kate has always had the right words to elegantly explain what I had a hard time conveying.

In August of 2017, my father was diagnosed with prostate cancer and I asked if Kate would accompany me. I watched her gently guide and comfort my family and friends when everything seemed so chaotic I was so grateful because she was the last piece in my puzzle and her interactions eased us through my dad's situation. She has a gift and my family instantly fell in love.

February 3, 2018 we were married. I was finishing up the last couple of months before my retirement. We were counting down the time on the island when in May, Kate's neck and upper back started giving her some trouble. We tried the chiropractor, to no avail, so she scheduled an appointment at Trippler Army Medical Center. The Doc ordered up some imaging and that's where I will leave you. Please enjoy my wife's book!

Life has dealt some pretty big blows in our lengthy 3 year marriage. We always joke that it seems like it has been 30 years since we said "I do." Kate can handle any situation and motivate herself to accomplish seemingly impossible tasks. Her super power is gracefully plowing and paving the untamed and treacherous path with her battle with cancer; she is a class act as you will soon read. My wife is phenomenal and I couldn't be more proud of her! I love you immensely Kate.

Grateful to God. Thankful for Kate's love and support, family, friends, Air Force, Tricare, numerous doctors, nurses, and all prayers.

Jim Cerny

STOP

*L*ate September 2013—Sleep and I had become distant friends. It seemed like I rested more than anything. I would fall asleep for what I would think was a decent amount of time only to look at the clock and realize it had only been fifteen to thirty minutes. That is what strong chemo does; you are more fatigued than ever before, but you have horrible insomnia. Getting up in the morning was a chore, but yet something willed me out of bed to stumble around. I was still in the early stages of my chemo regimen, and most of the side effects were controlled. Little did I know just how bad it would get.

That day, I got up and wandered in a fog into the kitchen where my husband and a couple of our employees were chatting. They were all getting ready to head out and begin their day on the ranch. After they left, I walked in circles as my inner Bully began to list off all the things I "needed" to do. I was overwhelmed by the list and the thought of the energy required to perform these tasks. Laundry, housekeeping, preparing for family coming to help, feed order for horses, client phone calls and emails, billing, exercise—the list and the voice continued in my head. I heard a running tally of all my failures, the reminder that I was going to get fat if I did not work out and eat right, and the you-shoulds and the you-betters.

Finally, I stopped, stood at the counter in the pantry, and yelled, "*Stop!*"

The voice was quiet for a moment. "*I can't!*" I cried. And in a moment of silence and clarity, I realized the only thing I had to do was take care of myself. I had three more months of chemo ahead of me, and I needed to learn to do what my body required, not what the Bully told me. I was thirty-seven, and that was the first day I listened to a softer voice, one that gave me permission to take care of myself in a gentle way, filled with love and compassion.

BEFORE

I believe I was born a perfectionist and learned at a young age the pleasure of praise. For me, the accolades from my parents meant I was worthy of their love. This then became the way I associated all love, being good enough to be lovable. This fueled my inner Bully. I never was good enough in my own mind but aspired to be perfect in every way, believing that I was fooling others and would someday be found out. The pressure I put on myself was immeasurable.

As I entered adulthood, I discovered a knack for business and self-employment. By the time I was thirty-two, I had owned four businesses and was starting my fifth. My last business endeavor had been affected by the recession, and I felt the failure deeply. I was determined to make my latest enterprise succeed.

My husband and I had recently purchased twenty-three acres and built our dream home as well as a barn with infrastructure for livestock and an extensive garden and orchard. I quickly accumulated a few horses of my own as well as boarding for other horse owners. This was my dream from childhood, and I could not believe I was living it. I pushed myself daily to improve my horsemanship as well as our accommodations. Marketing strategies played in my head, and I looked for ways to draw more people through my gate. Eventually, I was asked to train a client's horse and then teach her granddaughter to ride. I had found my real talent and strength as a horse trainer and children's riding instructor. I loved the combination of working with horses and children. As a result, this snowballed into a success I had not anticipated.

Despite the growing riding school and training program, I continued to think someone was going to reveal I was a fraud. My inner Bully fed on my fear and the pressure of business in the equine industry. I would wake at 4:30 a.m. as the Bully began the insurmountable list of to-dos for the day. I would roll out of bed, grab coffee, and begin my chores. I never thought of taking care of myself or slowing down.

I became "Commander Kate" to my husband and employees. I pushed myself and all those around me as if we were enlisted in the military. I heavily praised others' success but strove always to do more myself. As each project or goal was realized, I was already moving onto the next. I did not pause or appreciate what I had achieved, just demanded more of myself. No matter how hard I had worked, how long the day, or how much I had accomplished, every day ended the same. While I was cooking dinner, the Bully would begin the critique of all my shortcomings, what I had not done, and the foundation for tomorrow's list would begin.

I worked seven days a week this way or, rather, I *lived* seven days a week this way. I would take some time on Sundays to trail ride if it was not show season, but there was always a list and the Bully reminding me of what was next.

Within a couple of years, my marriage began to fall apart. We were business partners more than anything. My husband had become disenchanted with the life we had created and spent less and less time on the ranch and drank more and more when he was there. He was miserable. I detested him for not working as hard as I did and for not helping me more. I was a workaholic, and he was resentful. We were not the type to yell and scream but just spoke with venomous tongues. Two people unable to admit that it had been a good ride, but it was over.

As the wet winter of 2012 gave way to the spring of 2013, the Bully pushed me ever forward. I was maxed out on boarding space, the longer daylight hours were adding lessons to the schedule, and I had two horses in training. I also was trimming hooves for other horses and donkeys off the ranch one day a week. I drank coffee all day to keep my energy up. I thought the fatigue was just the result of my schedule and creeping closer to forty.

FIRST DIAGNOSIS

*I*t was mid-June 2013. The past two weeks had been a whirl-wind. I had gone in to see my doc about a rash that would not go away (ringworm). While I was there, they asked me to come in for a complete physical since they had not seen me in a while. I went back a couple of days later for the whole nine yards. The PA asked me if anything had changed. I mentioned the lump in my right breast but that my mother had fibroids, and I was guessing that was what it was. She then did the breast exam and ordered a mammogram and ultrasound. "Just to be safe." I think she knew it was not a fibroid.

I left the appointment and got in my truck. The tears came like a waterfall as the sinking feeling settled in. Something in me knew this was horrible. I needed support and called my sister Emily. I told her about the appointment through tears. I wanted her to give me some sort of assurance that the sinking feeling was wrong and all would be okay.

"Oh, sweetie, I'm so sorry. You know yourself better than any-one and are very in touch with your body. When you close your eyes and go to that place in your breast, what do you see?" Em asked.

I began to sob. "Oh, Em, it's horrible! All I see is black! It's so horrible."

She tried to comfort me and encouraged me to tell my husband when I got home. I did not feel ready. I needed time to process and prepare myself. I waited for a few days to tell my husband. I was surprised when he offered to take me to the mammogram and ultrasound. He kept a positive attitude about it and was convinced it was not cancer. I think the idea terrified him more than me.

The mammogram was clean, but the ultrasound showed several masses in my right breast. I could tell by the pity on the radiologist's face that I was in trouble. This was followed a few days later by a biopsy and five days of waiting for results.

It was raining the day I was supposed to get my results. My doc's office called as I was on my way to the breast imaging center. Although they did not give me any news over the phone, they said when I was done to come straight to their office and they would see me immediately. I knew then I had cancer.

Hearing those words, "You have cancer," is like nothing else. No other "bad" news felt anything like those words did. I had no control, knowing my body had betrayed me and something growing inside was trying to end my life prematurely. That tunnel is long and deep. I felt tremendously alone. People spoke, but I did not really care what they said.

The next step was by far the hardest, harder than the chemo- therapy would end up being. I needed to call my three sisters and my parents. For me, calling my parents is more than just Mom and Dad. There is my father and his wife, my stepmother, my stepdad and his wife, and then my biological mother. I am very close with all of them except my mother. She is mentally ill, and our relationship was more often strained and difficult than not. I feel blessed to have intensely close relationships with the other four of them. They are the people who raised me and have guided me through life. I called each of my sisters first. Em had an idea this was coming, but Sarah and Heidi were completely shocked. They had plenty of questions I could not answer other than to tell them what the next appointment was for and when. They instantly offered to come help however and whenever they could and tried to comfort me with their love. Next, I called my stepdad, Richard, and his wife, Sue. Sue had just finished her own battle with breast cancer a year prior, and they had just been at my house for a visit a month ago. They had a clear idea of what lay ahead for me and offered lots of support in ways no one else could. I waited the longest to tell my dad, Tom, and his wife, Mary Kaye. I knew that they were in the midst of a big fundraising weekend with their church and would be hard to catch until it was over. I sent a text message to Mary Kaye asking them to call me when it was over and they were at home together. I will never forget the moment the phone rang, and I knew it was time. I made sure they were sitting down, and then with a warrior's resolve, I said, "I have breast cancer." I clearly heard my father's heart break as Mama (my affectionate name for Mary Kaye) tried to hold both of their hearts together. There was silence as their tears began to form, and they tried to breathe. It was suffocating news. Like my sisters, they had questions I could not answer, but I told them what I could. They asked to call me back in a day or so, after they had some time to digest this information. These conversations were emotionally exhausting. The two or three days that followed the diagnosis were filled with sleepless nights, distracted days, and far too many hard conversations.

I dove deeper into my work to stay busy and avoid thinking about it in between the phone calls to oncologists, radiologists, the hospital, and other doctors I was trying to get appointments to see. I had constant anxiety that made me jump every time my phone would ring. The docs thought that it was caught early and was most likely early stage 2. All I wanted was it out of me. I weighed the various options—lumpectomy, partial mastectomy, and double mastectomy—and decided to have a double mastectomy. I did not want to have to go through this agony again.

It was about a week of waiting, pre-op consultation, blood work, and of course, working. I was consumed with the fear of losing all that I had built. The Bully fed on this fear and pushed ever harder for me to do more so I would be "ready." I was beyond exhausted as the cancer was feeding on my stress and fear, soaking up my energy and bringing me closer to an early grave. And yet, she pushed.

One last lesson, one last trail ride, one last day of hoof trimming. Surgery was on Tuesday, and I planned Monday for my personal prep. Sunday was my last day seeing clients off the ranch for at least a month. I was unable to round up any help and hit the road alone. It was a great day driving from one remote equine lover's property to the next. My final client's home was off a four-by-four road. I took my time getting there, enjoying the scenery and smells. I trimmed three horses for her and informed her of my situation but that I should be back at it in a month to six weeks. I headed home early in the evening, just wanting a drink and bed. It was done, the last of my horse work before my battle began. My mind swam in every direction. I turned off the radio and began a conversation with my breasts. I cried. I broke up with them as you would an abusive lover. "You are beautiful, and we have had a lot of fun together. But you are trying to kill me," I said out loud.

Sue had prepped me for what to expect from the surgery and gave me a sense of ease as I was rolled in and prepped. Surgery was early and took over six hours and revealed that the cancer was more advanced than they had thought. I had multiple tumors in my right breast, and over half of my lymph nodes were cancerous. A double mastectomy was the only option. This put me at stage 3C as far as they knew. I would be sent to Oahu for a PET scan to rule out any metastasis. I felt like someone had taken the lid off of the jar that contained my life and a vacuum was sucking it away. I just wanted that lid back in place and for there to be an end to all the bad news.

Through each step, Sue had guided me, giving me questions to ask and hints to help things go more smoothly. I never felt alone. She was full of advice and understanding. A couple of days after surgery, I called my family to tell them all what I now knew and update them on the next steps. When I told Sue the stage of my cancer, she said, "Sweetie, I'm sorry, but I can't help you. I will be able to help prepare you for chemo, but you are in uncharted territory for me." I know she was just being honest, but I felt like the lone soldier on the field. Her breast cancer had been stage two and found relatively early. She had undergone a double mastectomy with reconstruction, chemotherapy, and radiation. There were similarities, but I was climbing my own mountain; and no one could make me move but myself.

When I look back at how I approached my fight, I feel the need to apologize to myself. I woke up from surgery and started doing range-of-motion exercises with my arms. I was chomping at the bit to get discharged so I could get back to walking around the ranch and get healed up so I could get back to work. The Bully was driving my recovery. Just hours after being discharged, I participated in the local Relay for Life by walking the one-mile survivor lap. There was nothing gentle or nurturing about the way I was facing this challenge. It was all "Commander Kate."

A few days after surgery, Emily and Ella, my niece, arrived. They were a perfect distraction as I healed and had to take it somewhat easy. Ella was a little over a year old and so much fun to be around. We would walk down to see the horses with her in the lead, removing her clothes along the way and playing in every mud puddle she could find. She had no fear and would boldly put her little hands through the pasture fencing to touch and pet the goats and horses. They all seemed to know that they needed to be gentle and kind to this little human as they sweetly placed their muzzles within grasp. Em and I walked and talked, cleaned out my closet of all my low-cut dresses and shirts that I could no longer wear, and shared coffee in the morning and cocktails as we cooked dinner. Before I knew it, it was time for them to leave. It was a difficult farewell. We both knew that the hardest part still lay ahead and that I had so much yet to navigate.

Although my upper-body use was limited for a short time, I walked and did lower-body toning exercises. I told myself, *If I'm not going to have a rockin' rack, I'm going to have great legs.* The whip still cracked in my head, and I still pushed full steam ahead. On August 1, as I was recovering from surgery, I finally met with the oncologist.

The first time I met him, he walked in and without introducing himself, said, "This cancer is really bad. You know that, right?" Was this even a question! "Apparently, since you are the oncologist and you are saying that." I responded. He talked to me about the chemotherapy cocktail they would be serving and that it was the most aggressive treatment available. I was on board. "Hit this shit with all you've got, Doc! I'm going in with guns blazing!" I said with my toughest cowgirl voice. We got through all the details, and he handed me several papers about the various chemotherapies and walked me up to the front desk to schedule my first treatment, September 9th. It seemed so far away, and I wondered if we were leaving any cancerous cells unchecked for a month. Chemotherapy could not begin until I had the PET scan to confirm the severity of the disease.

I now refer to the combination of chemotherapy drugs I received as the trifecta. The first, Adriamycin, also known as the "Red Devil" for its red color and hellish side effects, is one of the strongest forms of chemotherapy used. The side effects include nausea, severe vomiting, diarrhea, hair loss, mouth and throat sores, thinning and weakening of finger and toenails, changes in color of finger and toenails, bone pain, weakened immune function, bruising and bleeding easily, pain and numbness in hands and feet, fatigue, loss of appetite, stomach pain or upset, menopause, joint pain, and heart damage. The second chemo drug in my cocktail, Cytoxan, was one of the original forms of chemotherapy that kills not only cancer cells but healthy cells as well and is associated with red and white blood cell suppression in bone marrow. The side effects are just as daunting as the Red Devil. Taxotere was also included, a chemotherapy that has been shown to be effective in treating breast cancer and shares many of the same side effects as the previous drugs, I did not focus on any of them. I heard little pieces of information and knew I would lose my hair, but I knew I needed to focus on other things, or the fear would send me spiraling.

Alone and still healing from my surgery, I took the interisland flight for my PET scan to find out if my expiration date was in the near future. Nervous and terrified and yet somewhat confident that they had gotten it all, I walked through the process. By the end of the day, I was home and anxiously awaiting the results.

The scan was done on a Thursday, and as I was leaving to see my surgeon for a postsurgical check the following Monday, he called with the results. I could hear the smile in his voice as he spoke. I was clean. No signs of metastasis. The lid was back on my life, and I could prepare for the next step of my fight.

I called my family members after I had a chance to meet with my surgeon. Finally, I had good news to share. A ray of light was cast into what had seemed like a bottomless darkness. I could hear the smiles in their voices and enjoyed celebrating this one small victory with each of them.

Chemo Begins

efore I could begin chemotherapy treatments, I had to have a power port placed in my upper chest. The procedure is a quick one-and-one-half-to-two-hour outpatient surgery. Luckily Dr. Pierce, the surgeon who had performed my mastectomy, was available and practiced in this procedure. I felt comforted to be working with him again. The port was placed on the left side of my chest, below my collarbone. I was very aware of its location and how it protruded from my bony chest. I quickly grew very self-conscious of people noticing it but knew it was a temporary and necessary part of my treatment.

My head had been filled with more advice than I could manage to absorb about preparing for chemotherapy. I held onto visualizing it as scrubbing bubbles and purple as a healing color, staying hydrated, multiple small meals, and being prepared for the myriad of side effects. I wore purple to my first chemo session. I took snacks, reading material, water, my laptop, and my headphones. I was told to wear a tank top so they could easily access my port for the infusion.

A nurse called my name and walked me back into the patient treatment area. I was weighed, and my vitals taken; then I was escorted into a crowded room filled with other cancer patients and showed to my recliner. With apprehension, I watched as they prepped the prechemo drugs, handing me pills to swallow, and then began the process of attaching the chemo pump to my port. The port gives direct access to a major vein; and therefore, any connection must be made with sterile equipment. The nurse pulled out the sterile pack that included the catheter that would lock into place over the port. After she had sterilized my skin around the port, she asked me to take a deep breath, and on the exhale, she pushed the needle through my skin and into the port. She then bandaged the area so it would remain sterile throughout treatment. After the premeds that were administered via my port had been given, two nurses dressed in special gowns to protect them from contact with the chemotherapy drugs began the first bag of the Red Devil. I had three bags of chemo to work through, each visit lasting eight to nine hours. As I sat there, the Bully carried on about me sitting all day, what I needed to get done when I got home, tomorrow and the next day, and getting fat—always getting fat.

Over twenty-four weeks, I had chemotherapy infusions two weeks in a row and then a week off. They administered half doses each cycle because of my size and sensitivity to the side effects. The first therapy left me feeling like my eyes were flat, and I noticed I was more easily worn out. The second left me with mouth and lip sores that would not stop bleeding because my platelets were too low. This was when I had my moment of clarity in the pantry and knew I needed to take care of myself and quiet the Bully.

The day after my second infusion, my sister Sarah and her son, Talla, came to visit. Sarah's husband had fought leukemia several years prior, giving her a clear understanding of what I was going through. The day that my lip and mouth would not stop bleeding, she knew exactly what to do. I laid down with ice on the sores for what seemed like an eternity to stop the bleeding. Her visit was not the relaxed time I had had with Emily. Instead, she cared for my side effects and took me in for my Neupogen injection two days after my infusion. This was given to boost my white blood cells that were being killed off by the chemotherapy. We did enjoy some nice walks together and visited for hours on the lanai; but the treatment was having an effect on my energy and appetite, and I could feel the nausea creeping in. Sarah knew so much about what I needed and cared for me with such tenderness. Her departure was difficult for me. I felt a bit stranded after she left.

After the fourth infusion, I could no longer control the nausea and fatigue. I quickly became bedridden and very sick. My oncologist and his nurses all emphasized the need to fight the urge to throw up as long as I could, but after the third infusion, I knew I would not be able to stop the inevitable. When the first wave came, I had no resistance left, and I fell into a pattern of increasingly violent bouts of vomiting that would leave me writhing in pain and exhausted. I felt like I had failed and was weak for giving in to the nausea, that all of this was happening to me and I was laying down and taking it. The Bully's voice was so venomous as she judged and critiqued everything I did or did not do. I had to get some relief in order to fight what was turning into a fight for my life.

With the fifth infusion, I had become extremely frail. I had nausea and vomiting, diarrhea, bone pain, and horrible abdominal cramping. Despite the best efforts of my oncologist and his team, my nausea was uncontrolled as was my pain. The vomiting would start on the way home from the chemo infusion and last for five to six days, giving me one day to collect myself and get ready for the next week's dose. The third week of each cycle brought great relief as I had it off and could catch my breath. I required assistance to walk any more than a few feet. I regularly required emergency fluids because of chronic dehydration as a result of the vomiting and diarrhea. The Neupogen injections were torture just because I had to get dressed and leave the comfort of my home.

In mid-October, my dad, Mama, and sister Heidi came for an extended visit. Heidi would be staying on for over a month to help take care of me and help out around the ranch. She was getting her degree in dietetics and had done some work with cancer patients. My nutrition was questionable at best, and her experience was potentially a key in getting me through the rest of the treatment.

They arrived the end of a treatment week before a week off, and we were able to enjoy some good days together. We even got out for some paddle boarding and a picnic. The next week, they all accompanied me to my infusion.

I had been taking CBDs to try to stimulate my appetite and aid in nausea control and the insomnia. I had been told to build up the dose and had doubled it the night before treatment. Although the amount of THC was supposed to be minimal, I woke up as high as a kite. It was a nightmare to be in a closed room (I now had a private room for my infusions) with the sound of the pump and all the sterile smells. Mama stayed with me, holding my hand in the dark as I slept my way through the entire nine hours.

Over the next few days, my parents saw my reality. They did everything they could to help me, even trying to get me to walk outside just to get a different view was too much. My father offered to lead one of my horses up to the house so I could see her and maybe that would help, but it was all in vain. I would have to vomit, or the pain would be too much. Then the next infusion came, and it was even worse. My parents' flight was the next day, and they left in tears not knowing if I was going to make it. They had never seen anyone so sick. Before they left, Heidi and Mama prayed over me. Them wanting to do this said all that was unsaid. I had doubted if I was going to make it through this fight.

At this point, I was about halfway through the treatment, and I had run out of the strength to keep going. I was so sick. I no longer had control over my bowels. The only nutrition I got was from liquid that rarely stayed down. I was unable to take care of myself in any way; I did not believe I had what I needed to keep fighting. I saw no light in my darkness. I began begging God to take me. I lay in bed all day crying from the pain and pleading with God to end my suffering. I just wanted to die. I did not have the strength to kill myself, or I might very well have taken my own life. I even contemplated the handgun that was in my closet.

As afternoon faded to evening and the daylight left my bedroom, I noticed the room become cloudy. My pain and nausea were suddenly gone. I felt as if I was being held like a child in the arms of a parent. I could not say that it was fatherly or motherly, but the best of both—strong and yet gentle, protective and openhearted, a mother and a father in one. I saw before me all those I had loved and lost. They stood at the foot of my bed with arms open and smiles that invited. I was overwhelmed with true unconditional love and a joy I had never known. Oh, how I wanted to go with them and be engulfed in these unearthly sensations, to be free of the pain, the fight, and the sickness. I was enchanted and ready to leave when suddenly I saw the image of my young niece and nephew and then my father writhing on the floor in tremendous emotional pain. I knew I was being given a choice, and without hesitation, I knew my answer. I wanted to stay to watch the next generation of my family grow, to be a part of their lives, and I did not want my father to feel the pain my death would bring him. Without a breath taken or word spoken, my pain returned, and I was back in my bed alone, suffering through a fight I now knew I would win.

HEALING

The rest of my chemo was not easy on me physically, but my resolve to finish drove me forward. Heidi was adamant that I find some additional help through acupuncture and any other means we could find. She all but carried me to my first appointment with an oriental medicine doc who specialized in cancer care. He was an angel. When he walked out and called my name, I feebly stood beside my youngest sister desperately hoping that this man would be able to give me whatever I needed to see my way to the end of this fight. He took my hands in his, looked me in the eyes, and said, "I am going to help you."

He worked to support my internal organs and body systems so I could finish chemo. He had so much knowledge and experience working with oncologists and the combination of chemotherapies I was on. He insisted that I finish the prescribed treatment plan due to the severity of my cancer. I drank a tea made from herbs on my weeks off and received acupuncture every week. Some of the side effects got better. I regained control of my bowels, and the diarrhea subsided. My labs started looking a little better, including my kidney and liver function. The pain and the vomiting were still uncontrollable and lasted through the two weeks following my last infusion. And then it was time to start healing all of me.

In all honesty, it took years. Chemotherapy had done damage to so many of my organs and taken so much life from me. Even though I was not receiving the infusions, it continued to affect my body for several months. I took an insane amount of supplements to help support my heart, kidneys, liver, spleen, and adrenal glands as they slowly healed. I had lost all stamina and a lot of muscle mass, so I started walking a mile every morning; and as time went on, the distance grew, and I no longer felt out of breath. I started lifting weights and grooming horses then feeding and doing chores around the barn.

Slowly, I felt more and more like myself again. I was stronger and could feel the progress I was making physically. I met regularly with my Eastern medicine doctor as we assessed the damage and long-term side effects. I had high blood pressure and had to take a low-dose statin. It became very clear about a month after chemo had ended that I had some major digestive issues. After eliminating most foods, eating a strictly alkaline diet and lots of testing, I was diagnosed with celiac disease. Adriamycin is famous, within the world of cancer, for leaving patients with either celiac or Crohn's disease. I felt lucky to have the prior.

I had a crash course in gluten and a gluten-free diet. As I began to eat the way my body needed me to, I felt better and better. I continued to work on the emotional aspect of all I had been through with daily meditation and journaling—healing my soul. Before I had been visited by God and my angels, I did not necessarily believe in God. I had been raised Catholic but never felt a strong connection through their doctrine; I asked too many questions and doubted many of the stories in the Bible. I was deeply spiritual and believed strongly in what I called the universe. An energy of sorts that was out there listening and assisting us if we were open to its messages. That all changed after my visitation. I found a faith in God that is unwavering. I can't help but weep when I talk about it and feel it in every cell of my being. I found different books to use as spiritual guides and worked to heal the emotional damage I had done to myself through the Bully.

It was incredibly difficult to dive into the damage done at my own hands. Slowly I felt complete love for myself, pride in who I was and what I had accomplished, and confidence in my ability to do whatever I set my mind to. I started each day with a meditation of personal positive affirmations. Hearing them in my head daily helped to keep the Bully at bay. I also journaled about what I dreamed for myself. My heart lifted, and I began to radiate positivity and self-love. I was so grateful to be alive. I still remember how sweet the smell of rain was, how exceptionally beautiful the sunrise was, how satisfying chores had become, and how joyful my entire being was. My threshold for suffering and sickness had become so extreme that life could not help but be seen through rose-colored shades.

About a month and a half after I had finished chemo, my father came for a visit. The last time he had seen me, I had been so ill he did not know if I would live. It was wonderful to show him the healthier me. To be able to do chores together and enjoy life. To laugh and cry together with cancer in the past. I treasured our time and the memories we shared.

After Dad left, I was intensely aware of a deep need to be with my family. Although they had come out to visit and help over the past several months, I needed more. I needed to show them that I was healthy again and how deeply I loved each of them. I ached to hold my niece and nephew and feel the life that had brought me back from the brink of death.

I spoke to my husband about making a trip to the mainland. As I had been finishing up chemo, he had proposed selling the ranch and moving to Panama. He had lived there for a short time as a child and had nothing but fond memories. As soon as I was no longer vomiting, the work began to get it listed. When I asked about visiting my family, he suggested that I wait until the ranch was on the market and then leave. Once it was sold, he would join me, and we could then move to Panama from there.

Now, as I write those words, I think how immature our thinking was—irrational dreams. At the time, I did not care. I just loved the idea of leaving. Getting away from the place I had fought the hardest fight of my life. The bed where I had risen time and again to walk to the toilet and vomit until I could no longer walk and then into a bucket. The hallway where I had lost control of my bowels for the first time. The sliding door through which I had watched the world, my world, without me in it. The weight of what had once been a dream come true was now a reminder of a living hell.

I made plans to fly into Utah in the beginning of July. I had a one-way ticket with the assumption the ranch would sell quickly and by summer's end, we would be heading south. I had intentions of spending time with parents, sisters, in-laws, and friends all over the western US including a family wedding in Montana. I basked in each moment I spent with those I loved and had missed so much. Living on an island had eliminated road trips from my travels, but I was able to take several during my sojourn.

I was free. Free of cancer, free of the ranch, free from the island, and free to wander. I hiked through mountains my soul had yearned for, drove through towns I had all but forgotten, and shared innumerable moments with so many people I adored. It was heavenly. Along the way, I was growing stronger and healthier experiencing life on the other side of cancer.

Throughout this time, the ranch sat on the market with very little action. It created stress between my husband and I and put additional strain on our marriage. He was growing bitter of me being away while he carried the load. As the days of summer gave way to early fall, it was time to plan my return. I would return to the island and the ranch in late October.

It was incredibly difficult to leave. I had never not wanted to go home, but this time, I ached to stay. The flight home was a mix of tears and sleep, and when I disembarked from the plane and stepped into the open-air terminal, the humid, sweet tropical air touched something deep inside of me, and I felt a new beginning. I was healed and ready to live the life I had left.

Eventually, I returned to teaching and training, but I wanted it to be different. The Bully was silent, and I no longer felt like I had to prove myself. I wanted to enjoy my work and honor myself. I did not want to trim hooves other than my own horses but was happy to teach others. I only worked four to five days a week and left the horses out in the pastures on Saturday nights so I could get some extra sleep on Sunday morning. I did not advertise for teaching or training and was very selective about the horses I took on for training, boarding, etc. I put myself first, and it felt amazing. I loved my work and felt good doing it, and it showed. I quickly had more students than I could teach, and somehow it all worked out.

The new and improved version of Diamond Valley Equestrian Center was everything I wanted. My students and their families were a part of me as much as I was a part of them. I took time for myself and was able to take better care of the horses and students. So much of my life was idealistic. However, it had become very clear to me that there was one piece of my life that was still not in sync with the me, I knew myself to be: my marriage. I knew it needed to officially end. I was back on my feet, healthy and strong, and we needed to stop pretending. I think there was a part of me that, despite carrying a broken heart, hoped that in mentioning the idea of divorce, he would want to save the marriage and love me the way I deserved to be loved. That was not the case. In a telephone conversation, I opened that door a crack, and before I could lift my hand from the knob, he was gone. The divorce was uncontested by either of us and took less than a week to finalize. Until the ranch sold, we would still have one knot left to undo. He quickly retrieved the majority of his belongings and moved back to the mainland. I was alone on the ranch.

I thought I had healed and that his leaving would bring closure, but it was just a beginning. It seemed that each day brought up a new wound that demanded my attention. I enjoyed being alone at the end of the day and having the time to work through so much pain. I felt physically rejected, deceived, played the fool, used, emotionally beaten down, and angry as hell. I slowly worked through all the parts of me that had been wounded in various ways over the years of my marriage. I was sure I never wanted to love again. I was done. Let me live out my life with my dogs and horses. Alone was so much easier. Besides, the idea of dating post-cancer was a mountain I did not want to climb.

It felt amazing to be successfully running the ranch on my own. Just the way the energy inside the house changed brought tremendous peace to me and all those who entered. My dogs were relaxed and happy. They went everywhere with me, and I loved it. At first, I was worried and scared that I would run the place into the ground, but my loved ones assured me that fear was based on messages I had been hearing for the past sixteen years of the relationship with my ex; and they were anything but true. I took on improvement projects on my own, protected the property from feral pigs, and maintained the home. Life was balanced.

I was so incredibly alive. I cherished the simplest of life's details and was truly grateful. My students and their families grew even closer. One of my adult students and I became close friends. She and her husband lived just down the road. I spent many an evening with them enjoying rich conversation and healing laughter. My days were blissful for a time. My heart healed, and the Bully stayed quiet.

DATING?

I had spent plenty of time alone throughout my life and had never felt lonely. I had enjoyed the time on my own and the quiet that it brought, space to think and listen to what I may not otherwise have been able to hear myself say. I always felt that this was healthy and an important part of maintaining balanced mental health. Loneliness is different.

For a time, the type of loneliness I experienced was deep and desperate. I was busy during the day, but the evenings, weekends, and holidays were challenging. Don't get me wrong. I had friends whom I would see for dinner, drinks, the beach, etc. It was not social interaction I craved, and it took me a while to realize what it was I really desired. And then one sunny beautiful Sunday morning while sitting on the lanai, crying for the aching loneliness I felt, it struck me: I wanted someone to love, and I wanted to be loved.

I had spent the time and done the work to heal most of my broken parts, and I was filled with love. I wanted to share that love with another person. I began to envision what qualities that man would possess, a list of what was important to me. Gone was the focus on the physical and superficial of my youth. This was a real man I wanted, a good man. I incorporated this into my daily meditation and asked God to help me find this man, the right man for me.

Finding Mr. Right was going to be a challenge for a forty-plus-year-old woman who worked and lived alone on a ranch, not to mention the breast-cancer piece. Just the thought of dating fed my long-quiet Bully. It was not my age, looks, financial or professional standing, or home but the history of the cancer and the fact that where once I had carried beautiful breasts, there now were two large scars. Actually, between cancer and injuries, I had fifteen scars from my collarbones to my hips. Who was ever going to want to look at that?

I turned to a longtime male friend who informed me, "Kate, you are so much more than tits. You are not looking for the guy that wants you for that. You are looking for a man who sees your substance."

He was right. The type of men I was looking to spend time with were not going to be like those I had dated twenty years prior. I also wondered, was I looking to fall in love or have fun for a bit on my way to love? I got a crash course in online dating and what site or sites were safe in my area, and I created a profile. Before I knew it, I was live. And the Bully continued to sleep.

Dating is scary and fun for most people. You are risking various levels of vulnerability, and it can feed your Bully. Depending on the type of area you live in, various factors play a huge roll in the experience you have as you get out and meet potential partners. Dating in a rural community on an island limits your options significantly. Don't get me wrong. I had fun, but my online dating experience was my friends' favorite form of entertainment. We would get together and laugh at the stories that either just came from messages that never got to a telephone call, telephone calls that were never going to result in a date, or the very occasional date that was not going to result in a second. There were a couple of men I went out with a few times, but they always ended up having nicknames that described why it did not continue.

Eventually, I took down my listing on the dating site. As much fun as it was, I got to a point where I was not enjoying myself. The wet winter was giving way to a sunny spring, and I had plenty of work to do. I refocused on my work, but one of the guys I had gone out with a couple of times had said something I kept hearing: "If you want to be able to move, why don't you sell your horses?" We had been talking about our dreams and desires, and I had mentioned that when the ranch sold, I planned to move to the mainland to be closer to my family. In hindsight, I was never really available to any potential suitor. I had no intention of staying on-island.

Sometimes people pass through our lives quickly but forever change the course we were on. There were several things that came from the brief encounter I had with the above-mentioned gentleman. We will call him Mr. H. He talked to me about vulnerability, selling my horses so I could pursue what was next and showed me a desperateness I did not know I possessed. As he spoke of vulnerability, he passionately described how liberating it can be when you allow yourself to let go and live without the fortresses we hide behind. He recommended Brené Brown and *The Power of Vulnerability*. I cannot overemphasize how powerful this book was in my life at that time.

I wanted to find love again, but I had never allowed myself to be vulnerable. I had been tough, guarded, and commanding in my marriage. Vulnerability had felt scary and therefore weak. Through the changes I had experienced as a result of my battle with breast cancer, I had come to understand the quick judgments we throw around based on our own insecurities. The voice who says, "Oh, what a bitch! She probably has a fancy car and a perfect house and, and, and"—meanwhile not knowing that she is married to a tyrant, those designer sunglasses hide the bruises, and her inner Bully is just as relentless as yours. I had realized that we all have insecurities and none of us are as we appear at first glance. Letting go of the isolation that my own insecurities had created brought me closer to living the life I wanted to live. Learning to risk without reward and be vulnerable absolutely set me on fire.

Mr. H was handsome and seemed to have a lot going for him. He appeared to be what I was looking for and wanted. I quickly fell back into old habits and did not honor myself, and the Bully arose. I allowed her to squash me to fit into his life so I would be more attractive because I was clearly not worthy or good enough. She hushed my calls to make me a priority and question inconsistencies in what he said or did. Slowly I grew smaller and more accommodating and yet resented him and began to withdraw. Luckily, this happened quickly, and I stopped seeing him. I was clearly not as ready as I thought. There was a desperation in my want to love and be loved, and that had given rise to the Bully and had me wading deep in insecurity and self-loathing.

Still I thought of selling my horses and the freedom I would then have to go and do. My heart broke at the idea of finding them new homes, closing up my riding program, and saying goodbye to my students and their families. Yet I knew it was the only way I could begin to live for me and find the life I was looking for. The ranch had been on the market for two years with no offers. I had relisted it with a new realtor and restaged it. I had no idea when or if it would ever sell. Twenty-three acres on the wet side of a rural island is not everyone's cup of tea.

Quickly I came up with a plan. I would have to turn the whole house into a vacation rental to support myself and move to another, more populated island so I could return easily until the ranch sold. It was doable but would be heart-wrenching. I meditated, prayed, and journaled about it. The voice of the Bully warned me of my failures and how I would never make this work. Despite my self-doubt, I knew this was the direction I needed to go.

I made the decision and began to spread the word around to my students and their families as well as my friends. On a Monday, I posted the news on social media, and within a week, my horses, tack, and supplies were gone. I cried myself to sleep every night as my heart broke. My horses had been my family. I had trained most of them myself and, in some cases, raised them. But I knew I was opening a new chapter, and it was time for me.

I called a friend who lived in the area of the neighboring island where I planned to move and made plans for a visit. This was the first trip I had ever taken where I made all the reservations myself, and it felt so good to have it all come together. I spent four nights there, enjoying a break from the ranch and a more beach-based lifestyle. I looked at rentals, hiked, swam, and enjoyed friends I had not seen in years. Before my return to the ranch, I secured a sweet spot close to the beach and down the street from my friend. I had a place to land. Now it was time to get myself, my two dogs, and the ranch ready for my move in one month's time.

A Fresh Start

As the days of my departure drew near, I spent time remembering and saying goodbye to every inch of the ranch. There were so many beautiful and happy times shared. I reminisced on the days that my ex and I had shared before it fell apart. The dreams of our masterpiece and all that we would do with the land. I recalled meeting so many people for the first time when they came to tour the facilities. The majority of them had become a part of my extended family, and I would miss them terribly.

I packed up everything as if it was going with me and planned to store it in the garage. I was moving with just the essentials. The house would be a vacation rental for others to enjoy until it sold. I knew I would return at some point but did not know when and wanted my personal belongings safe. On the day I was leaving, I walked to the top of the drive with the entire property spread out below me, and I spoke to the land. I thanked it for all the breathtaking sunsets and sunrises, for the fresh fruit and vegetables we grew, for the memories, and for dreams realized and lessons learned. And then I said goodbye one final time.

A dear friend drove my dogs and me, Albert and Moe, to the airport. I was filled with excitement and confidence that I was on the right path. The month of prep had gone very smoothly. My plan was to live on the neighboring island for a couple of years, hoping that the ranch would sell, and then move to a mountain town on the mainland, close to family. I wanted to have fun, play, date, travel, etc. So much of my life recently had been difficult and serious. It was time to kick up my heels and relax a bit.

Upon arrival, I grabbed the dogs and rental car and headed to our new home on the beach. We got there early afternoon on a perfect Hawaiian day. I unlocked the door and took my first steps into our new home. It was perfect, peaceful, and spacious with tall ceilings and large windows everywhere. I could hear the waves crashing on the beautiful sandy beach. I had very little furniture, but I had shipped over several boxes of my belongings I needed to put away. I blissfully organized and decorated my space. *My space*, just for me and my boys(Albert and Moe). We had taken the first steps in our new life.

Before long, I had met most of my neighbors, and the dogs had adjusted beautifully to our beach life. After about a week, I decided to test the waters and reactivate my profile on the dating site. Before long, I had a couple of dates set up. I planned to meet a guy on one of the beaches near my house one evening. We had texted and talked a bit previously. He had been forthcoming about having had a large noncancerous brain tumor. I took advantage of the moment to breach the subject of my breastless chest. I posed the following, "So I hope you're an ass man." The conversation easily led from there to my battle with cancer. He was not spooked, and we looked forward to meeting in person.

It was close to sunset when we met. I had Moe and Albert with me, and he instantly offered to take a leash. I was surprised by his comfort with them, and they both seemed to like him. We walked and talked, slowly moving along the beach as the sunset filled the sky with the colors only found in the tropics. We bumped into some of my neighbors and chatted for a bit. He was comfortable and relaxed, and something about him made me feel very safe. We walked back to his car, and he insisted on giving my dogs and me a ride home. It was dark, and he did not like the idea of us walking alone. So I agreed (I usually *never* would have let a guy know where I lived after only a short visit).

When I went to get in his car, he opened my door and did the same when we arrived at my house. He helped me out and made sure

I had both leashes before hugging me good night, at which point I made sure to gently kiss his cheek. I thanked him and headed into my house. He was sweet and kind and like no one I had ever dated. He texted me later that night saying that he had enjoyed our visit and would like to set up an actual date. We made plans for dinner a couple of nights later.

His name was Jim. He was in the air force, thirty-nine years old, from Iowa originally, never married, and had no kids. He had picked me up and taken me to dinner at one of the nicest restaurants on the north shore near my house. It was sunset, and we had an amazing view of the sun setting on the ocean from our table. I was impressed by his timing and wondered if it was intentional. The food was delicious, and the conversation flowed easily between us. Time stood still as we submerged ourselves in our own world. Still, when I think back, it was just us and the view.

Before our night ended, I knew I wanted to see Jim again. When I got home, I realized he was, by far, the most interesting, courteous, and thoughtful guy I had dated ever. We made plans for a second date that weekend. Before long, we were seeing each other at least twice a week. I was cautious and maintained my "me" time. I had found a small place to teach using the owners' horses and was enjoying my beachy horse life. I was not looking to fall in love and did not want to lose myself to another man. He put no pressure on me but made our time together count.

I had long since taken my profile down and chose to date Jim exclusively when I began to realize I was falling in love. We had been dating for a couple of months when my sister Sarah called to tell me her husband had just been diagnosed with a rare form of esophageal cancer. I took the next flight to be with them. It was during my time away that it became crystal clear how much I cared for Jim. I beamed when I talked about him and wanted to share everything I was doing and experiencing with him.

Jim did not have a lot of serious relationship experience, and he was a somewhat reserved guy. I knew I was going to have to be the one to risk and allow myself to be completely vulnerable by saying "I love you" first. I was absolutely terrified, but I had learned that without risk, there is no potential for gain. I had to trust and put my heart out there again. So, I wrote an eloquent email expressing my feelings for him and hit "Send."

He responded with, "Hello Love"…and I melted. Throughout all this, the Bully had been pretty quiet. She had reared her ugly head a little in the form of insecurity, and I had been able to shoot her down quickly; but my complete vulnerability had given her a door to walk through, and she moved back in. Her voice was small at first but grew as I continued to feed it. The constant message of "not enough" echoed through my head and drove my perfectionism. I had to maintain my body so Jim would not reject me. What if he figured out I was not as smart as he thinks I am? What if I screw up something for him professionally? I would second-guess and perseverate over conversations I had with his colleagues and friends. Critiquing my every movement, word, and behavior. Thinking how I could compensate for what may have been seen as inappropriate.

After we had only been dating for a few months, Jim's father was diagnosed with prostate cancer and had to have surgery. Jim asked that I join him for a trip home. I would be meeting his parents and staying in the house he grew up in. I was very nervous. I had met his sister and her family previously when they came to visit Jim a couple of months prior. We got along very well, but I had no idea what to expect from his folks. I tried to place myself in his mother's shoes. Jim was her boy, and here I was, the opposite of what she had most likely thought of for him. I had tattoos, was outspoken, strong, independent, divorced, unable to bare children, and hauling trunks full of baggage. Definitely *not good enough*! But, I put on my confident face and figured that they would see how I loved their son and hopefully accept me.

I have never felt more instantaneous unconditional love than I did when I walked off that airplane. Jim's mom hugged me like she was never going to let me go; she had loved me before we even met. The tears in her eyes and the smiles on both of their faces silenced the Bully. All that I thought was not good enough, did not matter to them. I loved their son, and they could see it. Over the next week, I spent loads of time with Jim and his family. We shared laughter and tears, stories and photographs, and love. Before we left, I was asked by his sister and mother what our plans were as far as marriage. I had fallen as much in love with Jim's family as I was with him and did not want to let them go.

So on a layover on our way home, once again, I risked, and I asked him what his intentions were. I explained that I felt connected to his family, as if I belonged, and needed to know where this was headed. "I plan to make an honest woman out of you," he replied with a grin, and my heart smiled.

We did not waste time. We were engaged that Christmas and married in February. I had no idea what being married again would do to fuel the Bully. She had moved in, unpacked, and filled my mind with all her self-abusive talk. Her voice had been building as Jim and I progressed through dating and became engaged, and once we were married and living together, the Bully used my fear of losing Jim to raise her attack. I was constantly aware of her berating me with "You are not good enough" or "You did not do enough" or "You're going to get fat, and then Jim will leave you. He will reject you and stop loving you." I lay awake at night replaying conversations and my interactions with everyone. I feared my rental on the ranch falling apart and failing as a businesswoman. The Bully had me convinced that somehow, Jim was going to see that I was not perfect and that would be the end.

PERFECTLY IMPERFECT

*B*y June, we were preparing for Jim's retirement from the air force and our move back to the mainland in August. Jim had accepted a position in northwestern Florida, working for a contractor at Eglin Air Force Base. He would start his new position in early October. There was a lot going on. The ranch was finally in escrow. We were buying a house in Florida, planning his retirement party, our wedding reception, and the trip that would take us and the dogs by plane to California and then by car, zigzagging through the continental US until we made it to our new home.

I was due for my annual check postcancer and made an appointment at the local military hospital. A friend of mine had died just a few months earlier from metastatic breast cancer, and I was on high alert. For the past few months, I had an ongoing pain in my back, next to my shoulder blade, that I had not been able to get relief from. I mentioned it to my new oncologist along with a pain in my left hip that had just started. He recommended a PET and bone scan. I scheduled both and expected them to be clear. The bone scan was done first and then the PET. It would take a few days to get the results, so I anticipated the "all clear" call early the following week.

"Mrs. Cerny, the doctor would like you to come in so he can discuss the results of the scans with you." The nice but firm voice on the other end of the phone sent me spinning. I felt sick, and a horrible darkness settled over me. She scheduled me for the next day. I began to sob as soon as I hung up the phone. I knew what that meant. There were indications of metastatic disease. The cancer was back. I was alone in our rental home. I fell to the floor and texted Jim to call me ASAP. I called the hospital back and begged to be seen that day. Jim called, and I crumbled. He would be home as soon as he could get there.

He found me in the hall, on the floor, gasping for air between the gut-wrenching sobs. "*No!* This can't be happening." Jim sat down beside me, and we held each other as we bawled.

We somberly drove to the hospital with tears in our eyes and our breath held. We sat beside each other, holding hands as the doctor spoke. From what the scans showed, I had a tumor next to my spine that was causing the pain in my upper back as well as a large tumor in my abdomen. "You have two years, maybe a little more." Jim's face contorted, and he wept with deep pain. I saw in that moment how much he loved me, a true unconditional love. It is tragic that it took this diagnosis and idea of an all-too-early death for me to finally see how deep Jim's love ran. Despite this moment of complete transparency, the Bully grew bigger as the doctor spoke.

I sat on the chair, no emotion. I steadied myself and breathed deeply. I had to be the example of strength. I knew everyone in my life would take the cue from me. I had to hold this ship together. Jim continued to shed tears as we moved through meeting the staff in the chemo room, the blood draw, and a barrage of information we did not yet know how to use.

A beautiful young woman sat across from me in the chemo room. She was bald from chemo, but her beauty superseded the side effects of her treatment. She kindly extended herself by sharing that she was fighting breast cancer. She did not know my history and was trying to be kind and comforting. She was easily ten years younger than me. My response was anything but friendly. "I had stage 3 grade C breast cancer five years ago. I was sure I had it beat, but now I have stage 4. I was just like you." I thought nothing of the interaction and continued to move through the process. I would later learn that my words had been crushing. I was the embodiment of her greatest fear.

I called my parents as soon as we got in the car. "This is the call I never wanted to make. There are indications that I have metastatic breast cancer." I tried not to fall apart and cry over the phone.

I wanted to be brave, to comfort them, so they would not hear my fear. I repeated this process with Jim's parents and eventually my sisters and close friends. I felt like every time I said "I have metastatic cancer," it was sealing my fate, solidifying the disease in me.

The first step toward treatment was an ultrasound to take a biopsy of the tumor in my abdomen. Something in me knew I did not have a tumor there. I had no intestinal discomfort, digestive issues, or pain. It made no sense that I could have a tumor several centimeters in length with no symptoms.

The days that followed were a blur. Phone calls to family, coffee with friends, long walks along the beach—anything I could think of to change the possibility of cancer. I stopped drinking alcohol. I was more strict about what I ate and added golden milk and CBDs to my health regimen. I also begged God to not let this be true. I cried almost daily. Jim was given the freedom to take whatever time he needed to be with me. I was never alone for an appointment. He took me in on the morning of the ultrasound. We waited for them to come get me and take me back for the procedure. When it was my turn, I kissed him and walked away; it would be a couple of hours before I was done. I felt strong and brave.

Once I was up on the table, they explained the procedure to me and helped me feel comfortable. They prepped my abdomen and began to look around with the ultrasound, comparing their location to the PET scan. They went over the area multiple times and could not find a tumor but saw that my intestine was twisted in that area. I was elated! No abdominal tumor! I strolled into the waiting area with a huge smile, catching Jim off guard. We embraced as I told him the news. We still had a long road ahead, but at least it was not as bad as they thought, and maybe, there was no cancer.

After the negative abdominal ultrasound biopsy, I was referred for a bone biopsy of the mass in my back. This was a tricky procedure due to all the nerves and potential for damage. In the midst of this time-sensitive measure, I also had planned a trip to the ranch to pack up what I had left behind and meet the movers.

The biopsy was performed on a Monday, and we met with the radiation oncologist for the results on Wednesday. I felt the dark cloud descending and that tug of intuition but brushed them aside and overcompensated by wearing a bright red dress for the appointment. It did not matter how big the smile was on my face or the prayers and pleading or the dreams of the future that filled my head. Cancer was looming.

The biopsy had confirmed that I had metastatic breast cancer. It was confined to my spine. Radiation would be used to treat the tumor growing beside C7-T2 as well as a mass growing inside C2 that would eventually pinch the spinal cord and kill me. It would take a month of five-day-a-week treatments. They wanted to start immediately, but it would have to wait a few days as Jim and I were leaving the next day for the ranch. Radiation would begin on Monday.

I had elected not to have radiation in 2013 and had no idea what to expect. Before we left the hospital, the radiation team took care of all the prep needed to begin the regimen. There was the tattoo placed in the center of my upper chest as a mark to line me up on the machine. Then a mask was made that would hold me in place and not allow my head, neck, or shoulders to move. It was made of a mesh material that was warm initially and cooled as it hardened. It was tight by the time it was done; there was no way I would be able to move.

That evening, Jim and I went for a walk, and I quickly began to fall apart as the reality of my situation began to settle in. The Bully was right. I was not worthy of Jim. I was so completely imperfect. Deeply flawed, how could he want to stay married to me? The Bully was beating me down. I was not enough by a long shot. Who would want someone so sick and basically dying? I was not the healthy, perfect wife Jim had married. I was going to be repeatedly changed as the disease took more and more from me.

"Babe, what's wrong?" Jim asked as he took my hand and saw the pain in my eyes.

"How could you want me? I understand if you want to leave. I'm not the woman you married just a few months ago. This is not what you signed up for. I'm not the perfect wife I wanted to be," I replied with tears streaming down my face.

Tears welled in his loving eyes. "You are perfectly imperfect to me. I'm not going anywhere. I love you, and we will face this together." Perfectly imperfect, and that was enough for Jim. His love was once again so apparent and unconditional. I felt safe. He was not going anywhere without me. We were a team.

Radiation

eing back on the ranch was a wonderful distraction. We had invited a few friends to join us for the weekend. Jim and I arrived one day before everyone else. I loved sharing with him what had once been such a sacred place for me. There was not much to pack up as I had left everything in boxes waiting for the day I would be ready to move. The weekend was blissful. We had a few things to take care of as part of the closing details, but the majority of the time was spent sharing the island, ranch, and time together. On Friday night, as we were all cooking and visiting, my radiation oncologist called to share more info from the biopsy. They had been able to identify one hormone marker, which meant they had a clear path for treatment post-radiation. This was excellent news! I shared it immediately with Jim and our friends. Hugs and tears were exchanged as we all breathed a sigh of relief.

Monday came too fast. We were back in our rental, and it was time to go for radiation. Jim would take me, bring me home, and then head to work. It was fairly simple, and the staff was amazing. The first two weeks of treatment went by without much effect. We were creeping closer to Jim's last day of work and the retirement party. My last day of treatment would be on the same day. His parents arrived to help me begin the cleaning process for our move that would take place the week after the party. I was feeling good when I picked them up and enjoyed visiting with them until Jim got home. The next day things took a violent turn.

Jim and his parents took me in for treatment. Everything went as it usually did. I felt major fatigue as we drove home and began to have some pain in my jaw. By the time we got home, I was nauseated, and the pain was getting worse. I lay on the couch with ice packs on either side of my jaw until I began to vomit. I was in rough shape from that day forward. I vomited multiple times a day every day and had the pain in my jaw for at least a week. The doc dismissed my nausea as being diet-related, but to this day, I believe that the radiation of C2 was interfering with my inner ear and making me sick. I also developed radiation burns on both sides of my neck.

I will forever be grateful for Jim's parents' presence through my remaining treatment and Jim's retirement party. In addition to taking me to treatment, they did most of the deep cleaning that needed to be done for us to move out of our home. Between the two of them and a small array of friends, I was able to host Jim's party. I remember still being sick from the radiation but knowing I needed to make the party happen. There was a mental fog that had settled in with the radiation sickness that I can only describe as having your brain cooked. I felt as if my head and brain were hot all the time. It was like I had been forced into a cave in my brain that I could still see out of, but only had a limited sightline. The whole world seemed dulled or muted, and my energy was fleeting.

Before we left for the mainland US, I had to begin part of what would be my treatment protocol for the foreseeable future. It was a two-part regime of hormone-suppressing injections and targeted pill-form chemotherapy. The first injection would be done at the hospital so they could teach Jim. He would have to administer two injections on our trip, one injection in each butt cheek. It hurt him far more than it did me.

The party was a success, and everyone enjoyed themselves. Within a few days, our house was empty, and we were on our way to California. We had a month on the road ahead of us with the dogs. We were excited for the adventure! The culmination of the trip would be a large reception hosted at his parents' country home.

Our journey took us zigzagging from south to north and north to south, taking the time to stay with family along the way. Jim had planned the trip and mapped out our route, keeping us mostly on small state roads and scenic byways. It was breathtaking. The dogs were experiencing so much and were far better behaved than I would have imagined. After three weeks on the road, we arrived in Iowa at Jim's parents' place. We would be there for a week prepping for the party and visiting with family and friends as they made it into town.

The day of the reception was unusually perfect. The weather had been wet and unseasonably cool, but it was sunny and low seventies that day. The whole day was beautiful. My family was there to celebrate and spent the day assisting in the setup before the party. The festivities got underway, and we were surrounded by family and friends, with their hearts full of love and joy. The day ended with fireworks and a huge bonfire. My heart was full, but my mind was distracted by the overshadowing of the next step in my treatment. I began the targeted chemotherapy that night, Ibrance, a pill that would work with my endocrine system to control disease progression in addition to the Faslodex injections.

After the guests had all headed back to their homes, it was time for us to hit the road again and make our way to our new home in Florida. We arrived on the thirteenth of September 2018, the day we closed on our home, a ranch-style house on a small lake in the country, space for the dogs, pine trees, and a relaxed lifestyle.

Dying

I wish I could say that I was at peace or happy in our new home, but I would be lying. I felt a dark cloud envelop me, and I was drowning in fear. Death loomed over me. The Bully had a new voice, and it was fueled by my dread. It reminded me constantly that I had a terminal disease. "Enjoy this Christmas. It might be your last" and other negative messages drowned out happiness and joy. There were also the images that would fill my head, of me wasting away surrounded by family. I kept thinking that if I just could figure out the right hoop God needed me to jump through, I would be saved. If I died, it would be my own fault.

Then there was the daily Ibrance and monthly Faslodex injections. The daily medication made me nauseated, and eating was anything but joyful. I took anti-nausea drugs like they were candy. Trying to drink enough water to avoid being constipated. Something inside me felt like this drug was not the one for me. There had to be a better way. The injections were torturous but necessary. Each syringe held 5 ml of fluid that was kept refrigerated until I arrived. Jim would warm the molasses-like fluid in his hands to help it go in more easily and then one syringe per butt cheek. I am not necessarily a meaty woman; therefore, there are not a lot of spots on my rump that were appropriate for these injections. Unfortunately, the right spot was on the side and to the rear slightly, just above my sciatic nerve. In January, the nurse accidentally hit my sciatic nerve and caused extreme pain to run down my leg for several days, in addition to the usual bruising and soreness I experienced with each injection.

Was this really living? Between the pain and the nausea, my quality of life was beginning to be questionable. I put on a mask and smiled to reassure everyone I was fine, but something in me knew I was dying.

That same month, I attended a yoga class and felt something pop in my back. I dismissed it and enjoyed the rest of the class. Over the next few days, I could not deny the pain in my back. For the next two months, pain would come and go, but I was forced to stop running. I was more easily fatigued and was diving deeper into depression as I was able to do less and less.

Meanwhile, Jim had decided to stop working and would be home more. He wanted us to have the time to travel and work on some home projects together. He finished up work in late March, and we headed off on a camping trip the next week. On the third day, we were forced to turn around and head home. I was in excruciating pain. I could not move without crippling pain shooting through my back. I could not walk without assistance.

After visiting the ER, we discovered I had a fractured vertebra. The doctor did not feel like that was causing the level of pain I was in. On Monday, I saw my oncologist, and he ordered new scans ASAP. I was forced to use a walker or wheelchair to move. Jim had to help me do everything. My doc tried all sorts of pain meds, and none of them worked. Some of them made me sick. Every couple of days, I was in and out of the hospital needing IV fluids.

The scan results were heartbreaking. The cancer had spread, and the medications were not working. I had lesions up and down my mid and low back, both sides of my SI joint, sacrum, and both hips as well as innumerable lesions on my rib cage and sternum, my skull, and four on my liver. I also had three fractured vertebrae that most likely would not heal.

Once they had the results, my team had to decide what the next step would be. What would be the most effective treatment to quickly stop the progression, and how could they get on top of the pain? It took a few days for them to make up their minds as they weighed the options. They had to consider how the cancer had adapted that would inhibit the effectiveness of various medications.

It was decided I would take a different, more traditional high-dose chemo in pill form and continue to take an infusion for bone density in the hopes of repairing some of the damage the cancer had caused. I was also referred to the pain management group in the hospital.

I cannot express the immense gratitude I feel for the doctors and nurses who became a part of my healing. For the first appointment, a consult, I needed my walker. During that initial visit, the doc was able to do an injection into the nerves on both sides of my SI joint, and I walked out on my own. It was an incredible gift. It had only been a month since I had walked on my own, but I had lost most of my muscle mass, especially my core. I felt weak, but willing. As I was checking out, the pain management therapist approached me and introduced herself. I will refer to her as Dr. P. She was very friendly and filled with positive energy. She said that she had read my case and was looking forward to working with me. *What?* I thought. *I'm not a fan of psychologists or psychiatrists. Y'all are nuts. My mother was one, and she's as looney as they come.* My internal dialogue carried on. I felt my walls rise, and I was ready to avoid this at any cost.

Over the next two months, my pain disappeared as the chemo and pain management treatments began to work. I was walking, although slowly, and working on putting myself back together physically. I was also seeing Dr. P every two weeks. Despite my resistance, I needed her. We unveiled the dark moments of my forty-three years, times of emotional trauma and pain, discovering toxic patterns in my relationship with my ex-husband, and my mother. Although both were damaging, those stories will wait for another time.

I realized so much through the healing work of old wounds and processing the Bully's abuse. It was painful and necessary. As I slowly cleared the muck from my past, I found myself wondering why I had not been aware of unconditional love. Why had I not felt that my father's love was unconditional? He loves me fiercely and would go to the ends of this earth if it would cure me of cancer. He would gladly trade places, and it pains him to be helpless in my fight. Yet somehow, I had been unable to feel or see it clearly.

We feel our parents' love through filters our mind creates when we are children. My mind saw him as the disciplinarian, the one I had to please. I saw his love as being conditional based on my behavior. I was blind to his active role in my childhood as my caretaker, protector, playmate, and first best friend. As this realization began to form in my mind, I had a glorious experience. In the midst of meditation, I was conveyed to my infant self, just born. My father was holding me for the first time (I am his eldest child). I could feel his strong arms gently holding me and his heart rapidly beating. Most importantly, I could feel the immense unconditional love and utter joy he felt in that moment. An eternal bond was created in that delivery room as he smiled down at my tiny face. I concluded, if we can let go of the filters, we can feel.

Knowing I had always been loved unconditionally propelled me forward in therapy. I learned how to quiet the Bully more permanently and reduce her power over me. As time passed, dying no longer filled my mind, and I began to focus on my future. I felt true joy again and could feel the biggest emotional wounds shrinking and the Bully getting quieter.

Eventually, I was able to identify whose voice was behind the Bully, what the ultimate message was that fueled the voice and chipped away at me. Like a record with a deep scratch, it repeated in my head, "Not enough. I'm not enough, not good enough, did not do enough, not worthy of love, not beautiful enough, not smart enough, not enough." Once I had digested the patterns and negative messages, I was able to replace the voice with my own: "I am enough, and whatever I do today is enough."

I am empowered by the healing this has provided for me. I have found my grace through learning to be kind to myself, forgive myself, and love myself unconditionally. This does not mean that the Bully's voice does not rise and that sometimes it even takes control. My fear rises when I am stressed or in the midst of change. Take for instance the first time my tumor markers rose. My instant thought was "What am I doing wrong?" And down the rabbit hole I went.

I was not only filled with fear but also with desperation. The truth is, I am always in a place of desperation, and that is what drives the majority of my fight with cancer. You never value life more than when it is slipping away. I want nothing more than to be told I am cured. Like so many other messages I have frantically searched for throughout my life, I look for it everywhere.

Although the cure I am searching for is related to my cancer, I easily stepped over all the "cures" I have found. When I started this journey, I was broken in so many ways, ways I did not even know. Over the past seven years, I have worked through and "cured" so many toxic emotions, patterns, and relationships. I have forgiven myself for the self-abuse and judgment. I have unearthed long-hidden secrets that ate away at me with their corrosive presence. I have discovered parts of myself I never knew existed. I have found a deep faith in God that guides and comforts me daily. Most importantly, I have learned to love myself unconditionally, being perfectly imperfect.

Thriving

*I*t is the beginning of September 2020, and my journey continues to challenge me in every way. This past spring, my oncologist started to see signs that the pill-form chemo was no longer working and referred me to Moffitt Cancer Center in Tampa, Florida. As COVID closed in on the US, I began the screening process for a clinical trial. After a couple of months of waiting and many trips to Tampa (a six-hour drive from my home), I started the trial drug. To this day, the cancer has not spread beyond the locations it had infiltrated in 2019, and the trial is working well—for now.

Although there were many serious potential side effects from the trial drug, I am experiencing almost none of them. I am healthy and active every day. I am filled with gratitude for the quality of life I enjoy and absolutely seize every moment. As a part of this clinical trial, I have a CT scan every six weeks; and every six weeks, I hold my breath. Sometimes it is easier than others to pooh-pooh my anxiety just based on how healthy I feel, but there is always a little voice second-guessing my resolve. I spend time wondering, *Is it still working? How long do I have? How many more options for treatment before I get really sick?* Something as simple as my liver values can send me tumbling down the rabbit hole of fear.

But from each trial comes triumph. I had been worried about some of the minimal side effects I was experiencing, such as hair thinning and my fingernails becoming weak and separating from the nail bed. Such small stuff, and yet my ego focuses on it and gives the

Bully fuel. "What will people think?" "People are going to stare at you." "Jim won't find you attractive anymore." After being worried that my latest scan results would show disease progression, I realized something: I would rather be bald and have no fingernails than be dead. It just does not matter. All the ways that we tell ourselves that we are not good enough really doesn't matter. Your wrinkles, gray hair, cellulite, muffin top, beer belly, acne, short legs, long legs, housekeeping, small breasts, parenting style, bald head, short or thin eyelashes, saggy butt, cooking—whatever it is that you pick on yourself for, *stop. Just stop!* You are enough just as you are today. For all the signs of aging that grace your face and body, there are thousands of people who wish they had the chance to grow old. For all your weight issues, there are thousands that would give anything to have a few extra pounds. And for every other complaint, there are millions who wish they had whatever it is you hate about yourself.

Love yourself just as you are, perfectly imperfect. Find your grace through kinder eyes and gentler self-talk. If it takes therapy to help you find it, then reach out and find the right person to help you. If that is not the path you choose, prayer, meditation, and feeling God's presence can be a significant source of strength and healing. Life is too short for us to torment ourselves and be unhappy. Start by listing all the things you are grateful for and let the first be *life*.

AFTERWORD

I don't deal well with being helpless to provide safety and to take care of those I love. But that's where I was, in Salt Lake City, on that beautiful early summer day, when Kate, in Hawaii, first called and told me of her cancer, her stage three breast cancer. The day vanished as I tried to understand what I'd heard and worked desperately to compartmentalize this new demon that had somehow insisted itself into my family, violating one of my children. A father's job is to provide love and safety, to be strong and protect the family, but I hadn't; I realized I couldn't.

Where to go from there…

Phone calls, visits, doctors, treatments, words of hope, talk of being finished, of healing. Then a second time and a third.

We've had those hard conversations about prognosis, life expectancy, conversations with clarity and tears. And Kate amazes me. She's the patient but her words and her attitude have challenged her circle of family and friends to drop the negative thinking, move away from that black hole. She doesn't need it, she'll be strong and positive and her strength supports all of us, those who know and love her, and we can give back, through our pain.

Tom Laabs-Johnson
Kate's Dad

CPSIA information can be obtained
at www.ICGtesting.com
Printed in the USA
BVHW032039110721
611670BV00022B/400

9 781636 924809